T0381377

KEMPE THERAPIES

Natural Remedy & Health Guide for Asthma, Arthritis, Cardiac, Cancer, Diabetes, Pneumonia, Whooping Cough and Other Illnesses

How Governments Could Save Billions And Work
At 20% To 50% Of Current Cost Levels
Non-Surgical Cardiac Approach
Non-Chemo Cancer Modality
Non-Pharmaceutical Diabetes Correction
Non-Pharmaceutical Blood Pressure Regulation
Non-Pharmaceutical Flu Remedy
Asthma Touch

Disclaimer
(to pharmaceutical industry)

Pharmaceutical products are tested to improve conditions -these tests are performed via double blind crossing modalities – with one pharmaceutical on one health condition the use of many different pharmaceuticals at the same time has side effects.

The outside interference with the body's health and immune system causes further weakness and requires thus more pharmaceuticals.

The dietetic answers improve chi flow to our organs and with the improved function less pharmaceutical can be prescribed.

The pharmaceutical industry should welcome topical products as they have no side effects and no contraindication.

It requires education in our society that antibiotic destroy bacteria in our digestive system and these have to be replenished as otherwise constipation is caused constipation causes the body to produce alcoholic substances.

The approach to generate food supplements which enable the body to improve its defences and heal itself is far superior as there is no influence to the defence mechanism of our body

http://perfection2010wins.ntpages.com.au
www.healthyairtoday.com
www.farabloc.com
www.454218.max.com

To order additional copies of this book, contact:
Xlibris LLC
1-888-795-4274
www.Xlibris.com
Orders@Xlibris.com

Alex Escobar:

'Gerhard, Nora and I talk about you as my angel and Nora's too. Your health analysis of my conditions when we first met just at my door and the advice which I followed strictly together with your treatments were pillars for my health.

'I was close to death, obese, with high blood pressure, overworked; and doctors told me I would require a kidney operation soon.

'Nora's blood pressure is normal now as well after following your advice and all without any pharmaceuticals.

'You assisted me as well, once I could not lift my arms. And you treated me for cardiac improvement. And within thirty minutes, I could lift my arms without pain'.

MEDICAL EXPLANATION

The indirect activation of glutathione production via energy field therapies (EFT), chakra, and meridian and acupressure and acupuncture, together with the dietetic food and food supplement–oriented catalyst approach regain body health, assisting the natural control mechanisms to take over again.

The cranial and muscular approaches allow correction, where required, to re-establish full chi flow (connectivity of nerves, ganglia, and body cycles and control mechanisms and metabolisms).

ACKNOWLEDGEMENT

Thank you to Mary Ann Meek and Guy Bennet, without them, I would never have learned kinesiology. Kinesiology courses visited in Brisbane were from 2003 to 2009 with teachers from Australia and USA.

Topical remedies were designed with experts in homeopathy Ruth Kendon

- PTSD (post traumatic stress disorder), stop smoking, addiction, migraine, headache, back pain, blood pressure, addiction, sinus, hay fever, bruises, swellings, muscle pain

- DV1 www.healthyairtoday.com, charged oxygen therapy, invention was manufactured first in Brisbane (pneumonia, whooping cough, skin disorders, intensive care wards, immune system improvement, catalytic use of negative charge on O2 (oxygen) molecule without production of O3 (ozone) – absolute no ozone production).

BIOGRAPHY

1960 - 1969 High School Ohm Gymnasium Erlangen Math Nat Science Gymnasium Most Special Subjects And All Common 6 Y Physics, 6Y Chemistry, 3Y Radio, 6Y Theatre, 3Y Newspaper, 6 Y Actor, 6 Y Quire , 3Y Special Quire, 2Y Public Speech

1969-1971 Banker Bavarian States Bank Finish Apprentice Ship after two years Best of Germany

1971 Chamber of Commerce Degree Banker Munich

1971 – 1975 Controller of petrol stations Elo R Kempe and selling kitchens and furniture Arzberger

1971-1975 MBA Commerce Law Banking Wuerzburg Univeristy Law, Banking, Insurance, Industrial Production, Revision, IBM Data Protection , Marketing Work Experience Siemens Neustadt Saale Optimize Production – US Army University Boston - & Degrees

1975 Financial Analyst Bankhaus Oppenheim M 1 M 2 M 3 Correlations to Share Market Correct prediction of BMW as purchase and German Market to soar

1976 First National Bank of Chicago Officer for business customers in commerce & industry with over 500 employees

1975-76 Type Writing Chamber of Commerce Cologne Degree

1976 Offer to work for Kingdom of Saudi Arabia $ 500 k

1976 Chamber of Commerce Degree Import and Export Merchant Cologne

1977 -1978 American Express Bank Officer Business Commerce And Industry North Germany Area Complete Duesseldorf to Hamburg

1978 Offer to become Chief of American Express in London in two years and leave for London now

1978 - 1994 Messrs R Kempe Erlangen CEO Wholesale construction materials , petroleum products Project Development Construction Gravel Pits Sales From 55 millions to 100 millions pa- Tenants Siemens Tengelman and other German Conglomerates

1994 Chamber of Commerce Degree to Educate Commercial Apprentices Office Business Administration

1996 – 1998 Project Development Shell Truckstop Pfalzfeld and Kirchheim unter Teck both turnkey projects

1999 -2014 Australia and USA RGF KEMPE and KEMPE Australia and Cleveland Visitor Villas Motel And DAIC LLC Kinesiology Courses 2002 – 2008 See Last Page

Invention of topical remedies home cooked remedies and non surgical cardiac improvement

www.healthyairtoday.com
www.farabloc.com
www.454218.max.com
http://xlibrishub2.com/wd/us/514040/author/
http://perfection2010wins.ntpages.com.au

SPECIAL KNOWLEDGE

How to cure most conditions with Kempe therapies acknowledged by natural therapy pages as new modality http://perfection2010wins.ntpages.com.au

This book may lead to new health clinic concepts, reducing costs by more than 50 percent.

Australian Kinesiology Association (AKA), the integrated new Kempe therapies are based on dietetic, chakra, chi, vertebrae, acupressure, acupuncture, and DV 1 (www.healthyairtoday.com) as well as topical remedies' development and their application points (homeopathic mixes of natural oils for migraine, headache, back pain, addiction, hay fever, sinus, stopping smoking, bruises, PTSD)

Knowledge to cure cancer and diabetes with a dietetic way discovery of left-right condition and how to improve the cardiac muscle without operation

Project developments with New Horizons Environment Finance Health

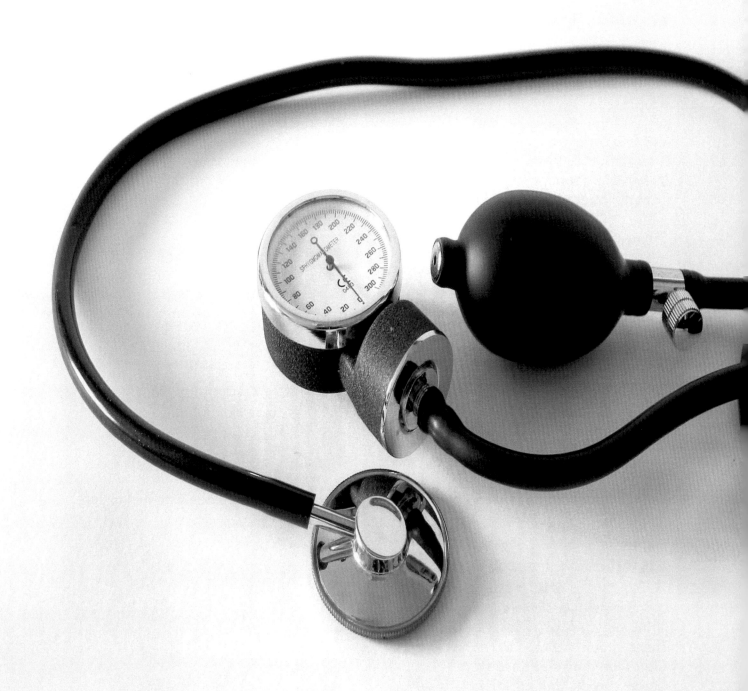

KEMPE THERAPIES
A–Z

ACUPRESSURE

'See what you can do for yourself'

Acupressure points are used to activate chi flow into organs.
Reflexology is using the end of meridians to stimulate body cycles and organs on hands and feet, and has been used for more than one thousand years.
Liver activation uses a point inside the left leg below the knee touch
At the same time, one of three points above the ankle, below the ankle, and halfway from the heel to the big toe on the left foot.

The point for cardiac activation is on the left hand.
• Walk with the right thumb underneath the little finger inside the left hand
• three thumb imprints underneath the ring finger and underneath the middle finger
• and use the last walking step as first of three steps down into the hand now you pulse
• Press rhythmic and activate the heart's chi flow

Reflexology is known for its success for one thousand years and more.

ACNE

Put 5 drops of tea tree oil (organic) in a glass of water and wash face with the mixture.

ALLERGIES

Clear the sinuses with sinus release (see Sinus Release).
Drink only boiled water (boiled chlorinated water).
There should be no cats in the house.
Clean the house of dust mites.
Clean carpets and curtains.
Treat skin with sodium bicarbonate and salt in bathtub (400g of each).
Inhale thyme (1 tablespoon of dried thyme mixed in 1 litre boiling water in large pot for inhaling).
Purify body with wheat-free diet, concentrate on vegetables (raw celery roots, beetroot, and carrots).
Detox with lots of boiled water, cooled (see also Hay Fever).
Skin attention with bicarb soda and water mix (see Dermatitis)
Have no cats in the premises where you live; coordinate left-right condition
Work on first, second, and third chakra and fourth chakra.
Complete reconditioning, re-correction.

ALZHEIMER

Magnesium, selenium, vitamin B12 complex, vitamin B2, chia (sage seed), vitamin C (ascorbic acid), turmeric, energy pill (best antioxidant)
No wheat, oats, nuts, raw red beetroot, cocoa, berries, grapes, milk thistle.
See also liver and kidney improvement and thymus gland and thyroid gland, atlas correction, muscular spinal correction (www.healthyairtoday.com).

ARTHRITIC CONDITION

Brush your body underwater in bathtub with 400 g salt and 400 g sodium bicarbonate for seven minutes. Include all parts of the skin. Shower first. Use bath more than 5 times. Skin assists liver and kidney to cleanse the blood and lymph (see also Liver). Drink sage tea (1 tablespoon sage with 1 litre boiled water).
Marinated onions recommended (marinate fresh-cut white onions in vinegar, honey, and olive oil; mix five to ten minutes before consumption). www.farabloc.com The farabloc blanket is reported to assist arthritic and osteoarthritic conditions with complete pain relief.

ASTHMA

Asthma touch stops coughing or asthma attack (my invention: light touch with three fingers on the inside of the arm underneath the wrist close to the outside of the inner arm, left or right). As you stop the attack, the asthma muscle stops growing and shrinks.
Clean house of dust mites.
Vacuum house, carpets, curtains, mattresses.
Clean air with sprinkle of 5 drops tea tree oil and glass of water.
Energy pill (www.454218.max.com)
Turmeric 5 g per day
Inhale thyme (1 tablespoon of dry thyme poured over with 1 Ltr boiling water) and drink thyme tea
No cats in the house or close by.
Use DV 1 (healthyairtoday.com and healthyairtoday.com.au)
Thyme: Add 1 tablespoon to 1 litre boiling water. Drink and inhale with towel over the head above pot.
Tea tree oil: Pour 5 drops into a glass of water, sprinkle in the air of room structure.
Excrements of dust mites: vacuum house, curtains, and mattresses; clean house and cupboards.
Inhale DV 1 (www.healthyairtoday.com).
Sinus attention urgent re-establish sinus defence system (if the sinus remedy is not available sniff in and blow out saltwater into both nostrils one at a time).
Sinus relief is one of my topical remedies. You use only 1/2 teaspoon with a glass of water. Sniffing in and blowing out from each nostril clear sinuses and activate tissue to full function again.

ATLAS correction DIY (Do It Yourself)

Move your head over the bed, lying on your front so when the head falls down the chin does not touch the bed. Breathe in deeply and slow so the shoulders raise and breathe out with a sigh, fast, with the head loose facing down and the chin not touching the bed. Repeat five times.
Test whether completion was achieved by lying front downwards and with knees bent. See that feet are on level and not in an angle and at the same height.

Correcting atlas and vertebrae—feet positions—therapy muscular correction:

     Lying supine on the chest with arms beside the body
     Knees bent so the feet are beside each other

There are possible formations:
     Left foot higher than right
     Both even
     Right foot higher than left

     Left sole towards right
     Right sole towards left
     Or outside, which is rather rare

     All those conditions are attended with an outcome
     Feet looking flat upwards and in level to each other

     To place correction in spot memory and base memory requires attention as well.

     The primary achievement is executed with breathing out.

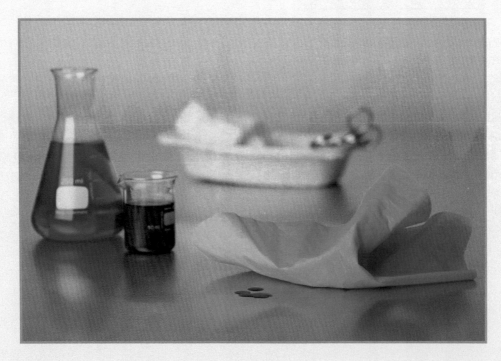

BACKPAIN

Apply peppermint-oil on fingertip. For perfect results, order Backpain Topical from Kempe Therapies (http://perfection2010wins.ntpages.com.au) 50 ml at $55
Spread elbows backwards at different height; engage in stretching exercises for the spine.
see also neck stress and shoulder stress relief

BIRD FLU

Infections cannot take place in the rooms that are secured by charged oxygen. www.healthyairtoday.com not only improves the immune system to resist the virus attack but also kills micro-organism so they cannot affect you. Once infected, we recommend the flu remedy (see Flu Remedy).

BLADDER

Bladder improvement with pumpkin seeds—meridian and acupuncture and acupressure. The seed of the pumpkin works wonders to the bladder. Also, melon seed should be consumed. Other treatment methods for the bladder are meridian and chakra and acupuncture and acupressure.

BLOOD PRESSURE REGULATION

Consume boiled garlic - take it out of the boiling water when soft - you may also drink the water.

BLOOD PRESSURE

High and low blood pressures are regulated by eating boiled garlic.
To get low blood pressure higher, eat rosemary (2–5 leaves per day).
To lower blood pressure, eat 3–5 dry juniper berries per day and comb back in S-curves from over the shoulder to below bottom with the back side of fingernails from left to right and right to left with 300 g of pressure—upwards and downwards

BRAIN TUMOR

Alkalize the diet with coconut cream and coconut milk. Place DV 1 close to the entrance of the respiratory system, with 300 mm distance from head (www.healthyairtoday.com).

Concentrate the diet on starchless products; only raw red beetroot, raw carrots, and raw celery roots.

Perform an atlas correction: Activate body with energy pill or use these ingredients: turmeric, grape seed, broccoli seed, red wine activant, selenium, zinc. Stay away from microwave cooking and put away electromagnetic waves close to the bed where you sleep.

Have Farabloc blanket around head, forming a faraday cage so that electromagnetic influences are shielded off.

BRUISES SWELLING MUSCLE PAIN

Peppermint oil on fingertip apply to bruised area. For perfect results, check http://perfection2010wins.ntpages.com.au. It costs $55 per 50 ml, which is more than two hundred applications.

BURNS

Instant application of emu oil pure (reported to lower degrees of burns by one, if applied within thirty minutes after the accident). For old burns and scars, we recommend Kempe tissue rejuvenation cream, also known as Kempe facelift cream.

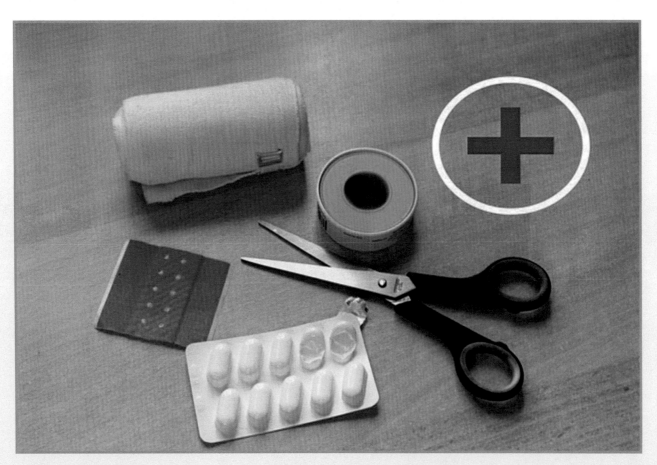

CANCER TREATMENT

Increase chi flow (see page 3) with muscular spinal and atlas correction and left-right correction placed in memory (acupressure inside hand and feet, acupuncture, meridian, and chakra work).
Drink 3 litres liquid per day (boiled water and then cooled)
(GREG FARREL HAD NO MORE CANCER OPERATION REQUIRED)
SIX WEEKS WATER, RED BEETROOT, CARROTS AND CELERY ROOT , NOTHING ELSE
Alkalize the diet with coconut cream and coconut milk. Place DV 1 close to the entrance of the respiratory system, 300 mm distance from head (www.healthyairtoday.com). Concentrate diet on starchless products; only raw red beetroot, raw carrots, and raw celery roots.
Perform an atlas correction. Activate body with energy pill or use these ingredients (turmeric, grape seed, broccoli seed, red wine activant, selenium, zinc). Stay away from microwave cooking and put away electromagnetic waves close to the bed where you sleep.
Have Farabloc blanket around body, forming a faraday cage so that electromagnetic influences are shielded off. NO MICROWAVE FOODS -

CARDIAC

20 minutes
The short-way approach goes straight into action on the cardiac after the balance left-right condition was corrected and leg length and foot position cleared; with the cardiac cranial test and if the slightest error or imbalance or resistance error comes up, correction is at place. The fast way requires correction in memory after correction and positive test . . .
Count and 100, 98, 96, 94, 92, 90, 88, 86,84
or sing a song,
Touch cranium above ear (and slightly more back approximately three fingers away from ear).
If no firm hold, improvement has to be performed.
Opposite of sing or count is to 'hammer' chest and back with 300 g–450 g flat fist or hand.

Cardiac danger is indicated by un-symmetric face, lips, and mouth appearance (left and right end of the mouth are not in level).

I can only emphasize on the clear warning of a stroke or a cardiac attack when this danger sign occurs. It requires immediate complete cardiac treatment to avoid severe complications.

The other alternative to a treatment is a cardiac test and operation to prevent the worst to happen.

Cardiac Improvement (No splint operation required; pacemaker to come out David Noah, Greg Farrell—Green Slopes Hospital. Alex Escobar's testimony: 'I could raise my arms without pain again and felt well'.)

The fact that the cardiac muscle was able to perform well again after appropriate cardiac cranial treatments could be breathtaking for the future of medical cardiac expenses in our society.

Just think of costs for pacemakers and pharmaceuticals after the surgical impact (blood thinners and other balancing medications required).

The Cardiac Improvement

Cardiac improvement is available as shortcut and complete body re-correction; if approached as shortcut, the slightest weakness acts as indicator and requires the appropriate correction and after the correction to be placed in memory.

The more safe way is the complete approach: test of left-right condition, muscular correction of spine and atlas, test of cardiac improvement requirements, cardiac improvement and placement of corrections *in memory*.
(Test of all vertebrae positions and correction and correction in memory.)

Test of completed left-right correction (foot position and leg-length correction):

Atlas correction, cranial improvement, and cardiac improvement as well as placement in memory.

Increase chi flow with muscular, spinal, and atlas correction and left-right correction placed in memory: acupressure inside hand and feet, acupuncture, meridian and chakra work.

Drink 3 litres liquid per day (boiled water and then cooled).

The shortcut is recommended only for patients who had a complete correction done once before within the last six months.

Even so, to this date, there was no patient with placement in memory showing symptoms that the old condition did re-occur without an accident. The test should always be performed.

Do Your Own Cardiac Improvement

Meridian

Movement starts with the right hand, fingers close to each other two inches outside the body.

Above the body (if you are lying down on your back) or in front of your body (if you are upright position).
Move from above / in front of the left breast nipple. Go up keeping the distance to the shoulder alongside the left arm inside and out on the ring finger of the left hand.

Cardiac Improvement Acupressure

(Assists even during transport to hospital for cardiac operation. Ten cases did not require operation. No case report which required operation.)
Walk with right-hand thumb imprint on your left hand underneath the bottom phalange of your little finger, three thumb imprints till you are underneath the bottom phalange of the middle finger and three thumb imprints down counting the third before as the first down. Once you go to the point, press in rhythmic way to create chi energy to the cardiac muscle.

Dietetic Cardiac Improvement

Dietetic Cardiac Improvement
Take B 12 Vitamin complex and magnesium supplements to clear arteries and veins and take 1/2 teaspoon of apple cider vinegar on a glass of water twice a day

COLON AND DIGESTIVE PROBLEMS

Vanilla ice cream and desiccated coconut, as well as coconut cream (natural), or coconut milk (natural) with milk products accelerate digestion (add coffee powder if coffee taste is desired). To line the bowels drink two cans of coconut cream per day. This also alkalizes the body.

CONSTIPATION

Eat vanilla ice cream with desiccated coconut, coconut cream and coffee powder and cracked black pepper and or chilli flakes.

CRAMPS AND SPASMS

A lack of magnesium causes cramps and spasms. Take magnesium supplement.

CYSTIC FIBROSIS

Meridian and chakra work to activate base chakras and main meridians (see Thymus Gland and Thyroid Gland), the enhanced chi flow—nerve connection—blood flow and lymph flow will carry away the dead cells and activate the body's defence system.

Vitamin B2 is recommended as well as B 12 complex with vitamin B6. For diet, 30 per cent of meals should be raw red beetroot, celery root, carrots. Wheat should be compensated with corn products

To reduce acidity and enhance alkalizing, avoid coffee and alcohol and replace with coconut milk, coconut cream, and cocoa drinks and replace sugar with honey. Farabloc blanket www.farabloc.com and www.healthyairtoday.com as well as flu remedy to enhance and support immune system.

DEMENTIA (see ALZHEIMER)

DEPRESSION

Hot dark chocolate, dark coverture chocolate, honey, atlas correction, exercise, breathing techniques, singing, music, gospel, swimming, diving, dancing, laughing gas, sex with spouse, beach walking, and coffee in moderation (www.healthyairtoday.com or www.healthyairtoday.com.au).

DERMATITIS, SKIN DISORDER. INFECTION, ECZEMA

Pamper on affected areas the following mix 4 tablespoons sodium bicarbonate with 1–10 litres water.

For complete body bath use 400 g salt and 400 g sodium bicarbonate if possible brush skin with low pressure.

Soak in mix of salt, sodium bicarbonate, and water—the weakness of the self-defence system is overcome, and the skin is able to perform its protective function without irritation again

DIABETES

Chi flow improvement: 10 g cassia per day (block electromagnetic fields)
Farabloc cage building solutions – dietetic answer cassia –
Spinal correction and others in memory—change electromagnetic fields
Farabloc blanket

DIARRHOEA

Sip Coca-Cola using coffee spoon also called teaspoon (recommended for all ages) efficient within one to a few hours.
Drink hot cocoa or chocolate after you stopped running to the toilet and have some salt chips.

DISKS

Regrow disks with 1 kg fish oil per day or 50 g chia seed and a tablespoon
Of flaxseed oil and grape seed oil (soak chia or sage seed in a glass of cooled
boiled water).

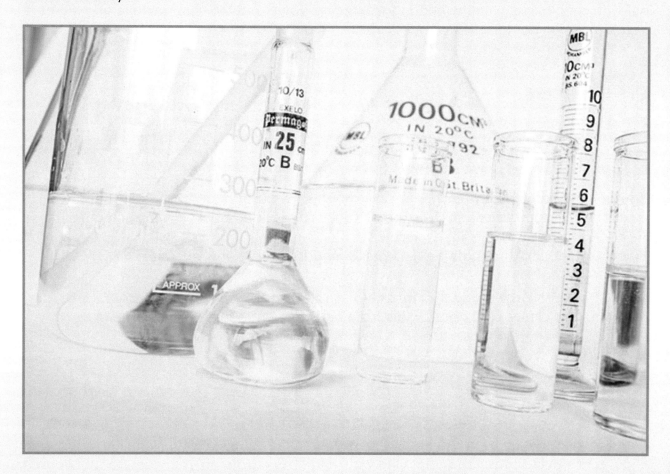

ENERGY

Lack of energy is overcome by exercise, swimming, vitamin B complex (double dose
the first day), the special aging Q10, selenium, cassia, walking, DV 1 charged oxygen
(www.healthyairtoday.com), blueberries, vitamin C in form of ascorbic acid, green tea,
sage tea, chia or sage seeds, grape seed, poppy seed, broccoli and broccoli seed,
turmeric ,chilies, pepper, cocoa, sex, onions (the doctor of liver), 3 litres boiled and
cooled water per day, bio-flavonoids, red beetroot, raw carrots, celery roots, singing,
praying (see also Depression).
Energy drinks V, Red Bull - Energy pill see end of book – how to order …

EXERCISES

Atlas Correction DIY (Do It Yourself)

Move your head over the bed, lying on your front so when the head falls down, the chin does not touch the bed. Breathe in deeply and slow so the shoulders raise and breathe out with a sigh, fast, with the head loose, facing down and the chin not touching the bed. Repeat five times.

EYE EXERCISE

Three years after I wrote the essay, the Cambridge University confirmed improvement of 1/4–1/2 di-optrin per week.

You don't need glasses after one or two months! Two hours per day, do the following:
12 circles, 12 points on each circle point, look forward and backward far, medium, close
12 circles horizontal and 12 circles vertical
Pigeon effect: look through the fist has nothing to do with this exercise!

On 12 vertical circles and 12 horizontal circles, look forwards and backwards, far, medium, and close. One hour of this training is known to improve the eyesight.

SHOULDER AND NECK STRESS

Do you remember the last time your neck was sore and stiff?
Here is the way to treat yourself: Place yourself against a wall with the head and shoulders staying pressed against the wall. Walk forward with your feet about two and a half feet, 600 mm – 750 mm – the pressure on neck and shoulders from the wall – increases as the angle position increased, stop after 18 – 23 seconds, stand upright, roll shoulders forward and backward. Move elbows outward at different positions and... done... cheers.

FIBROMYALGIA

Fibromyalgia is a disorder caused by vitamin B2 deficiency. Take vitamin B2. Improvement is rather instant (memory, sagging tissue, nerves). Sage tea is also recommended as well as chia seed (sage seed). Complimentary farabloc blanket should be used www. farabloc.com.

FLU REMEDY

Improve your immune system. This recipe has assisted thousands to **fight flu within twenty-four hours** without antibiotics.

INGREDIENTS:

1kg honey, five brown peeled onions, 10 tablespoons olive oil, 1/2 coffee spoon or teaspoon dry chilli flakes, 2 cloves garlic (the whole garlic round).
Use a flat frying pan. Separate 3 litres water.

PROCESS:

Boil 3 litres water and cool in the fridge ready to drink.
Cut peeled onions and garlic to 1/4-inch pieces, pour olive oil in frying pan, add chilli flakes.
Sizzle mix till onions turn from white to glazy. Take off heat. Pour 1kg honey over mix. Test with fork that garlic and onions are soft. Consume once cold with cold water. Your body will flush out (a mild diarrhoea is caused) and you will sleep after six to eight hours. You are close to fit again.

GALLBLADDER

Increase chi flow with muscular, spinal, and atlas correction and left-right correction placed in memory: acupressure inside hand and feet, acupuncture, meridian, liver, and chakra work. Drink 3 litres liquid per day (boiled water then cooled)
Infection: Drink sage tea and camomile tea (1 litre boiling water on 1 teabag)
Stones: Place aluminium bowls three sizes one at a time over gallbladder area
Above right hip, beat with teaspoon, tablespoon, long wooden spoon. Soundwaves will tremor the stone. Grape seed oil will assist to pass the stone fines (ten tablespoons grape seed oil).

THE HANDSHAKE

Touching the other's hand with a handshake might already talk and tell a lot about the health condition of the person: arthritic deformation of fingers, cholesterol swollen back of the hand (showing arteries and veins full of effluents) in case both or one of these conditions is present you act.
For arthritic pain, we recommend 400 g of sodium bicarb and 400 g of salt in a bathtub with water and brushing the skin for seven minutes—all areas of the skin underwater. For cholesterol and to clean veins and arteries, take magnesium supplement and two B12 complex vitamin pills with lots of water a day. To activate the digestive system, use vanilla ice cream with desiccated coconut and coconut cream if wanted with coffee powder. To activate the liver use boiled or marinated onion.

And to activate the kidney, we take the 3 litres of water sage tea a day (water boiled and cooled in fridge).
Never take water from the tap for drinking. Boil it first as otherwise, you may get allergies due to chlorine.

HAY FEVER (See SINUS RELIEF)

Clear sinuses by sniffing up and blowing out saltwater. For prefect results,
use Sinus Relief $55 for 50 ml (http://perfection2010wins.ntpages.com.au).
Effective within seconds after one application.

HIGH BLOOD PRESSURE

Eat three to five dry juniper berries per day and comb back in S-curves with the back side of finger nails.

IMPOTENCE

Impotence is cured with melon seeds, ginger root, kambudscha, rhino horn, chillies, pepper, camomile. From Bavaria we know about Sauerkraut with beer or white wine. Other methods are acupuncture, acupressure, and meridian work as well as hand two feet above first chakra and charge up see thymus gland.
Sex drive cured with melon seeds and lemon seeds, turmeric, and vitamin C. Other methods are music and massage.

INFECTIONS

The following deficit of supplements would weaken the body to get (ready) for infections: zinc (metal), vitamin C (vitamin), magnesium (metal), salt (mineral), green leafy vegetables (bio-flavonoids). Loss of blood, diabetes, wrong nourishment, especially not enough salt or not enough water will cause the deficit to influence negative on the health side.

Skin disorders, pneumonia, infections of the respiratory system, sexually transmitted diseases—even airborne infections will take over the body as the immune system is too weak to perform.
To boost the immune system fast, we recommend salt and the flu remedy (see Flu Remedy)

INSECT BITES OR STINGS

Fresh-cut onion placed on the bite/sting/venom area. Place front and back of onion cuts and use four to seven onion slices for immediate relief. Repeat as long as pain or swelling persists.

INTESTINE

Increase chi flow with muscular, spinal, and atlas correction and left-right correction placed in memory: acupressure inside hand and feet, acupuncture, meridian, and chakra work.
Drink 3 litres liquid per day (boiled water then cooled)
After antibiotic, the replenishment of bacteria is required with special yoghurts.
Ulcers are treated with bismuth. Balance is achieved with coconut cream.
Sensitive to alcohol and drug abuse (too much acidity balanced with 1/2 teaspoon sodium bicarbonate with 1 glass of water)
Increase chi flow with chakra one and two treatment as well as energy complexion with hand over navel with knees-up position

KIDNEY

Increase chi flow with muscular, spinal, and atlas correction and left-right correction placed in memory: acupressure inside hand and feet, acupuncture, meridian, and chakra work.
Drink 3 litres liquid per day (boiled water then cooled)
Infection: drink sage tea and camomile tea (1 ltr boiling water on 1 tea bag) (antibiotics)
Stones place aluminium bowls three sizes one at a time over kidney area
Above right or left hipp – beat alu bowls with tea spoon – table spoon – wooden long spoon
Sound waves will tremor the stone – grape seed oil will assist to pass the Stone fines (10 table spoons grape seed oil)

LEFT-RIGHT CONDITION
Intensification

Repeat command:
Hold the forehead
Rest
Patient trains alone or with family member

I asked a doctor in the hospital with over forty-five years of experience as GP, 'What was your most challenging experience in life in your work?'
He answered, 'Whenever we did everything by the book but it didn't work'. I said, 'Yes, that's what you call the left-right condition when the body mixes up left and right in it's sub-conscious mind and thus cannot heal itself in alpha wave because left and right is mixed up. Kinesiology calls the correction "balance"'.

To test whether the body has a left-right condition, the patient is asked to lift and stretch out limbs (legs and arms) together and a cross. If the command is not followed, without hesitation, by mixing up left and right, intensification is achieved by the patient repeating command before the lift or the practitioner holding the forehead and or short rest. Also the patient can train with family members at home. The cranial touch after correction of the left-right condition and the muscular spinal correction is achieved by holding one arm and fourteen positions above the patient's body, starting from the upper legs over the back side and on to the spine while holding a pressure and command against the calve muscle of the left and the right leg. Whenever the muscle testing is weak, a rub with knuckles of the hands beside the spine with above 300 g of pressure enables the body to correct and the muscle to hold against pressure after correction. The correction is placed in memory intermediate with the cranial touch and the hip bone across and later place in memory by holding the stretch out arms one at a time when eyes are closed and looking up and looking right and looking down and looking left. With the correction, new ganglia patterns are formed, and the body is able to heal itself again as the left and right condition is overcome and corrected. It is quite usual for patient to pass out and sleep when the left-right condition, the spine, the atlas as well as the cardiac muscle are corrected in the same treatment. The patient does not recognize this passing out or sleeping time and has a feeling as if the treatment was only five or ten minutes instead of the one to one-half hour it takes.

Severe cough condition prevailed after three months visiting health practitioners in Australia.

Bio-flavonoids, salt, and DV 1 (www.healthyairtoday.com) treatment under DV 1 device
Work was performed with DV 1 connected to electricity close by.
'I cannot get rid of my cough for six months now and went from doctor to doctor'.
The girl was in her twenty-plus years and looked devastated. The left-right condition was present, and the vertebrae as well as the atlas did require correction. On top, she showed kidney stress with the white in the eye centre pupil shadow. I mixed up a cocktail of boiled water, salt, and pine needles (the long ones) in the blender and asked her whether it tasted okay. She loved it and took 80–120 ml and some water thereafter.

After the treatment, I requested her to cough as severely as she could. She could not cough anymore!

Why would salt and pine needles help such a lot with the body in the reactive positive mode?

Remember salt is even injected as saline solution in cases where no blood is present during operations and surgeries. It says, 'You are the salt of the Earth'. And pine needles contain bio-flavonoids as substance.

The importance of bioflavonoids is not noticed by many doctors, however, as important as supplements of vitamins (C, D, A, and B group), metals (iron and zinc—carriers of oxygen inside our body), and enzymes.

Omega fatty acids (sage seed and fish oil krill) and other substances (selenium and calcium) are important and vital to our body organism

Just to deposit calcium into our bones or to the skin tissue, plenty of vitamin C and calcium have to be present – ideal supplied by celery and apples (remember the saying 'an apple a day keeps the doctor away'). Please note: After the menopause, the female body does not break down calcium from cheese or milk as it did prior to the menopause. Apples and celery are recommended to replace the cheese and dairy products.

LIVER

Increase chi flow with muscular spinal and atlas correction and left-right correction placed in memory (acupressure inside hand and feet, acupuncture, meridian, and chakra work)
Drink 3 litres liquid per day (boiled water and then cooled) The onion is the doctor for the liver!
Consume boiled or shortly fried onion it must still be white and not brown fried when you eat it. The colour should be glazy. The liver can be improved with meridian work: acupuncture, acupressure, lots of water, no fat, no alcohol, no constipation (the body produces alcohol when slow digestion is in progress). The acupuncture treatment of the liver once assisted me for the gamma gt values from 134 to 68 within ten acupuncture treatments three days apart.

Another patient's gamma gt reading improved from 120 to 44 just with acupuncture and onions. What a surprise!

LOW BLOOD PRESSURE

Rosemary herb (eat two to three rosemary leaves per day, dry or fresh)

LUNG CANCER

Alkalize the diet with coconut cream and coconut milk. Place DV 1 close to the respiratory system entry 300 mm distance (ewww.healthyairtoday.com and www.helathyairtoday.com.au). Concentrate the diet on starchless products; only raw red beetroot, raw carrots, raw celery root, and water.

Cancer diet: raw red beetroot, raw carrots and raw celery root, boiled water (cooled, warm, or hot)

LUNG PNEUMONIA

(www.healthyairtoday.com) and inhalation of thyme steam
Lutheran Church testimonial was for three patients who stopped pneumonia within two to three days with charged oxygen therapy

LYMPHATIC DISORDER

Cassia 10 g per day and energy pill (click join on www.454218.max.com - choose cellgevity product)
Energy pill consists of a multilateral body stimulus natural supplements (grape seed, turmeric, milk, thistle, etc.) both taken together will be able to stop lymphatic pain within two to three days.

MENOPAUSE (FEMALE)

Oestrogen complexities after menopause are solved by cranberries and apple and celery, replacing the dairy products as milk and cheese for calcium intake cannot be absorbed after menopause unlike before menopause.

Minerals are in spices and root vegetables.
calcium (bone structure, skin) , salt (infections), selenium (memory, cancer, psoriasis, autism), zinc (inflammation, infection, autism, cancer), magnesium (joint pain autism), iron (beef) (all body functions)

MIGRAINE

Use migraine relief http://perfection2010wins.ntpages.com.au
$ 55 per 50 ml, more than 100 applications

Otherwise, use atlas correction and peppermint oil on fingertip on temple and below ears and as stretch on the neck from left to right. This will stop migraine development within seconds.

MULTIPLE SCLEROSIS (MS)

The nerve infection of the spine is caused by a virus, which can only be killed with bismuth, a toxic metal (see your doctor), selenium, lysine, B12 complex, energy pill, honey

NERVES

Caraway seeds mixed nuts and raisins, selenium, lysine, celery, and apples (min 300 g per day), coverture chocolate, (cocoa powder alkalised with dextrose for drinks), hot cocoa, honey

ORGAN SPECIFIC IMPROVEMENTS

Meridians and chakras as per 3,000 years old teachings
Acupressure points and reflexology
Vertebrae correction to solve chi flow impairments
In case of virus activity inside the body, think of antibiotic and bismuth as assisting metal supplement but only as prescribed

The fact that the cardiac muscle was able to perform well again after appropriate cardiac cranial treatments could be breathtaking for the future of cardiac medical expenses in our society.

Just think of costs for pacemakers and pharmaceuticals after the surgical impact (blood thinners and other balancing medications required).

PANCREAS / DIABETES

Increase chi flow with muscular, spinal, and atlas correction placed in memory
Diet of 10 g of cassia per day

PNEUMONIA

Three members of the Lutheran Church in Mt Cotton were cured from pneumonia within three days with the Device DV 1 www.healthyairtoday.com
connected to electric power in 0.5 m - 1 m distance from the head.
Members of the Seventh Day Adventist Church, Cornubia, with a thank you for the Samoan sarongs presented to me and Mary Ann, I still remember the warm welcome in the Seventh Day Adventist Church and the sincere attitude when listening to my experience and the detailed question and answer session, which assisted many Christians of the church to improve their health and remember the numerous long-lasting conditions including shoulder issues, which were treated with good outcomes in consequence.

WHOOPING COUGH   www.healthyairtoday.com

DV1, www.healthyairtoday.com, was invented to create micro-organisms-free room air structures, which benefit humans and plants and animals and devastates micro-organisms. Per ccm, more than ten million extra electrons on molecules and 02 (oxygen) but not 03 (ozone) are produced! The charged oxygen enables the body to perform tissue healing in an air-structure with reduced micro-activity – infection free for airborne infections.
We distinguish between tissue healing inside the respiratory system, inside the body and outside for skin health; the device delivers health for both tissue systems.
For babies who cannot take medications and suffer from whooping cough, DV 1 is the answer to improve their health (www.healthyairtoday.com).
Connect the device to electric power and have the baby's head in 600-800mm distance.

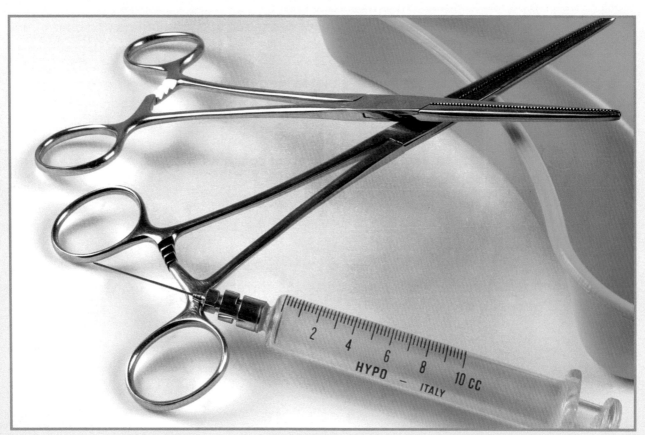

PREGNANCY

During pregnancy, more rest is required as well as plenty of calcium and vitamin C (apples, celery, cheese, milk) and fish oil as well as krill and sage seed (chia), vitamin B complex, and zinc, music, singing, dancing (classical music), swimming as favourite sport and bath (pool or bathtub) before going to bed so the foetus can place itself in a comfortable position without the weight as its weight is carried by the water. Please reduce the intake of coffee or alcohol as both will lead to miscarriage or too-early birth. To start giving birth, a pumping pulse with the thumb inside the hand(s) will assist giving chi energy to the uterus. Minimum 1,200 g of beef per week for the iron required. (See also Liver, energy, and energy pill.)

PREGNANCY EXERCISE

Prior to giving birth, exercises from breathing to vertebrae and taichi and yoga are recommended. The position for breathing exercises should be standing or lying down in giving birth position.

PREGNANT SLEEP

To allow the foetus to place itself comfortably prior to sleep, have a bath in a bathtub or in the pool or just lie in the water. As the water carries the mother's body, the stress in the uterus and foetus disappears and a comfortable position can be found. It is imperative for a pregnant woman to take plenty of calcium and vitamin C (apples, cheese, celery, and milk should be 15–25 per cent of the diet). If there is an allergy during pregnancy, use bicarb soda and water. Drink chlorinated water only after boiling it.

Have tea of papaya in case of uterus infections. Boil papaya leaves with water and flush it in the uterus using a devise. If papaya leaves are not available, use four tablespoons of bicarb soda in a bucket of water and flush in uterus and take a bath as well with 400 grams of bicarb of soda in a bathtub of water.

RHEUMATISM

Drink 3 litres of sage tea per day and see arthritic condition. Follow recommendation for liver and kidney in this book.

PSORIASIS
Inside salt, zinc, Q10, B complex, no wheat, red beet root, greens, leaves, biofllavonoides, pine-needles, selenium
Outside bath salt sodium bicarb; DV1; +immunesystem-yoga-prayer; meditation

Inflamed ganglia connectivity or ganglia action with short circuits, virus infection boost immune system with flu remedy, charged oxygen therapy (www.healthyairtoday.com)

SHOULDER AND NECK STRESS

Here is the way to treat yourself: Place yourself against a wall with the head and shoulders staying pressed against the wall. Walk forward with your feet about two and a half feet 600 mm – 750 mm – the pressure on neck and shoulders from the wall – increases as the angle position increased, stop after 18 – 23 seconds, stand upright, roll shoulders forward and backward. Move elbows outward at different positions and... done... cheers.

SINUS RELIEF

Clear sinuses by sniffing up and blowing out saltwater. For prefect results, use Sinus Relief $55 for 50 ml (http://perfection2010wins.ntpages.com.au). Effective within seconds after one application.

SKIN IRRITATIONS

DV 1 (www.healthyairtoday.com) in 600mm of irritated areas connected to electricity and skin area exposed to room air as well as a bath in sodium bicarb water.
On one bathtub use 400g or sodium bicarbonate. Place irritated skin in bucket with bicarb of soda and water . Improve immune system with flu remedy.
Fungi as well as rashes and other skin irritations disappear with the treatments mentioned above.

SKIN DISORDER

Boost immune system (see Flu Remedy)
Zinc, Q10, calcium, vitamin B 12 complex, and vitamin E

Celery, apples, DV 1(healthyairtoday.com), bath sodium bicarbonate and water (300 g–400 g bicarbonate soda and salt in bathtub) brush skin 7 for seven minutes, all parts, including head. If no bathtub is present, wash affected areas with water and salt mix and bicarb of soda mix.

Use antibiotics for viral infections.

SLEEP APNEA
(sleepless nights, problems waking up, or trouble sleeping)

The calcium cycle in our body deposits calcium where required most; if not in the bloodstream, calcium is taken out of the bones and deposited on to the skin tissues or broken bone. As long as vitamin C and calcium are present in the bloodstream, sleep is not disturbed. To achieve enough calcium and vitamin C in the bloodstream, the consumption of apples and celery is recommended. 'An apple a day keeps the doctor away'.

We recommend 300 g of apples and celery sticks as minimum intake especially prior to sleep as it is during the alpha wave that the body repairs itself.

SMOKING AND HEALTH SUPPLEMENTS

Studies have shown that not only do vitamin supplements fail to lower cancer risk, but they can actually cause cancer—most notably, the 1994 Finnish study found that smokers who took beta carotene, which the body converts to vitamin A, actually had a higher risk of lung cancer than men who didn't take the supplements. We recommend no smoking as tobacco changes body functions.

STOMACH

Increase chi flow (see page 2 and page 3) with muscular, spinal, and atlas correction and left-right correction placed in memory: acupressure inside hand and feet, acupuncture, meridian and chakra work.

Drink 3 litres liquid per day (boiled water and then cooled).

After antibiotic, the replenishment of bacteria is required with special yoghurts.

Ulcers are treated with bismuth. Balance is achieved with coconut cream.

Sensitive to alcohol and drug abuse: too much stomach acidity is balanced with 1/2 teaspoon sodium bicarbonate with 1 glass of water Increased chi flow with chakra one and two treatment as well as energy complexion with hand over navel with knees-up position. First chakra treatment, see Thyroid Gland: (hand two feet above area between navel and below), fingertips together with "tent" over navel.

STRESS IN THE EYE

Father Marce, the most confident father and priest I have ever met, showed stress on the eye. His lids were closing his eyes in and there's a white cloud inside the iris—the eyes centre—kidney alarm. An appropriate treatment was applied, and the eyes were bedded in white surroundings again. The stress on his kidney was gone as there was plenty of water to drink and his smile was even brighter than before the treatment. Certainly, we got a lot of work done to celebrate a re-organization of the community by receiving permission to place St Mary statue inside the cathedral at St Matthews.

SUPPLEMENTS

All these work as antioxidants in our system:
For omega fatty acids: chia (sage seed), fish oil, krill
Body functions: grape seed (enzymes), sage seed, broccoli seeds, melon seed, milk, thistle seeds (liver, silymarin), chilli,
Corriander intensifies peripheral blood circulation (Alzheimer, memory loss)
Pepper cracked, Muscat grape seed, nutmeg, turmeric, paprika seeds
Garlic, ginger, kambudscha kava (anxiety), sage (as tea anxiety)
Parsley activates kidney function, pumpkin seed (bladder)
Cassia (diabetes), Sauerkraut (fermented cabbage), and white wine or beer for potency (sexual erection for male) thyme (respiratory system), camomile (nerves), nuts (neurological and nerves), oats (nerves and energy), onion (liver)

THYROID GLAND

Upward move alongside main meridian in front and back activate the under-functioning gland.
Downward move alongside main meridian in front and back reduce overactivity.

Under and over chi regulations and over-functioning of thyroid gland is addressed with a calming meridian activation in front of the body and behind the body, in the centre of the body with a movement to a two inches distance from head over the spine towards L-vertebrae (lower lumbago) in front towards the navel and beyond. Three movements every four hours. Dietetic: nuts are recommended
Other recommendations are aromatherapy and lavender oil in under chi, which means the thyroid gland requires improvement in the function; spinal and atlas correction, meridian improvement in front of the back or the front in the middle with two inches distance from areas along the sides of the spine towards head and out movement over the head. Five movements every three hours. Dietetic recommendation is to eat seeds of hanf also called canary seeds or seeds of marijuana and seeds of poppy and to take flu remedy in order to boost the immune system.

THYMUS GLAND

Upward move alongside main meridian in front and back activate the under-functioning gland.
Downward move alongside main meridian in front and back reduce overactivity.

Under and over chi regulations and over-functioning of thyroid gland is addressed with a calming meridian activation in front of the body and behind the body, in the centre of the body with a movement to a two inches distance from head over the spine towards L-vertebrae (lower lumbago) in front towards the navel and beyond. Three movements every four hours. Eat nuts use aromatherapy and lavender oil in under chi, which means the thyroid gland requires improvement in the function, required spinal and atlas correction, meridian improvement in front of the back or the front in the middle with two inches distance from areas along the sides of the spine towards head and out movement over the head. Five movements every three hours. Dietetic recommendation is to eat seeds of hanf also called canary seeds or seeds of marijuana and seeds of poppy and flu remedy.

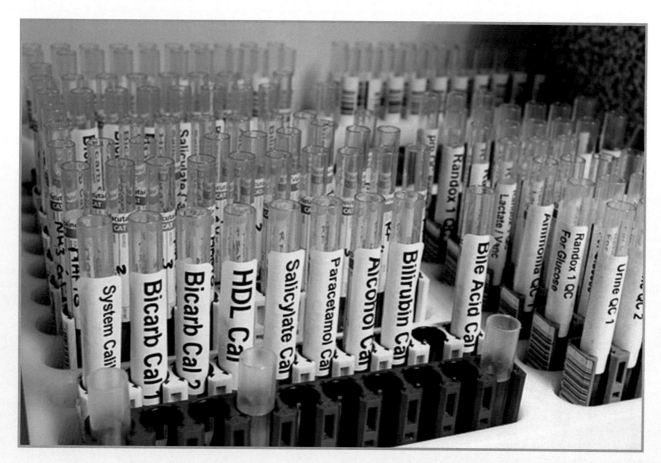

Tissue repair external

Apply Kempe facelift crème (removes wrinkles scars and enhances tissue repair) from www.healthyairtoday.com. Vitamin B12 complex, coconut cream, coconut milk to drink. Emu oil creme or Emu Oil improves the skin tissue in case of burns.

UTERUS INFECTION

Have tea of papaya in case of uterus infections. Boil papaya leaves with water and flush it in the uterus using a devise. If papaya leaves are not available, use four tablespoons of bicarb soda in a bucket of water and flush in uterus and take a bath as well with 400 grams of bicarb of soda in a bathtub of water. Improve immune system (www. healthyairtoday.com; salt, flu remedy).

VERTEBRAE CHI ACTIVATION EXERCISES

Elbows out to different height positions from down completely to hands above head, the elbows whipping outwards, back, and forward (remember the duckling dance).

VERTEBRAE IN POSITION

(Lynn Noffke: Leg length correction: 'I did not require a hip operation anymore'.

VITAMINS

The body can absorb vitamin A from the carrot only when fat is present (butter recommended). Too much vitamin A can create health hazards.

There have been reports that vitamin A overdose is possible and can have harming effect to the body especially for lung cancer.
Vitamin B complex is known to revive the energy cycle and cleanse veins and arteries when certain B vitamins are present (B6 and B12) .
Vitamin B2 recommended is for fibromyalgia
Vitamin C is known to assist in preventing and fighting cancer conditions required for the calcium body cycle essential vitamin in the form of ascorbic acid – requires constant Input as body disperses of it in a two- to four-hour cycle
Vitamin D formed by the sunlight and skin; deficiency could cause harm
Vitamin E: too much of it increases the blood pressure essential for body functions and energy

WEIGHT LOSS

Completely leave wheat out of the diet.
Drink a glass of boiled water cold with 1/2 spoon apple cider vinegar twice a day.

Wrinkles

Kempe facelift crème and Kempe wrinkle crème for eye zones

ZYSTIC FIBROSIS

Meridian and chakra work to activate base chakras and main meridians (see Thymus Gland and Thyroid Gland). The enhanced chi flow (nerve connection) blood flow, and lymph flow will carry away the dead cells and activate the body's defence system. Vitamin B2 is recommended as well as B complex with 12 B Vitamins – dietetic 30 per cent of meals should be raw red beet root , celery root , carrots – wheat should be compensated with corn products
To reduce acidity and enhance alkalizing avoid coffee and alcohol and replace with coconut milk, coconut cream , and cocoa drinks and replace sugar with honey. Farabloc blanket www.farabloc.com and www.healthyairtoday.com as well as flue remedy to enhance and support immune system.

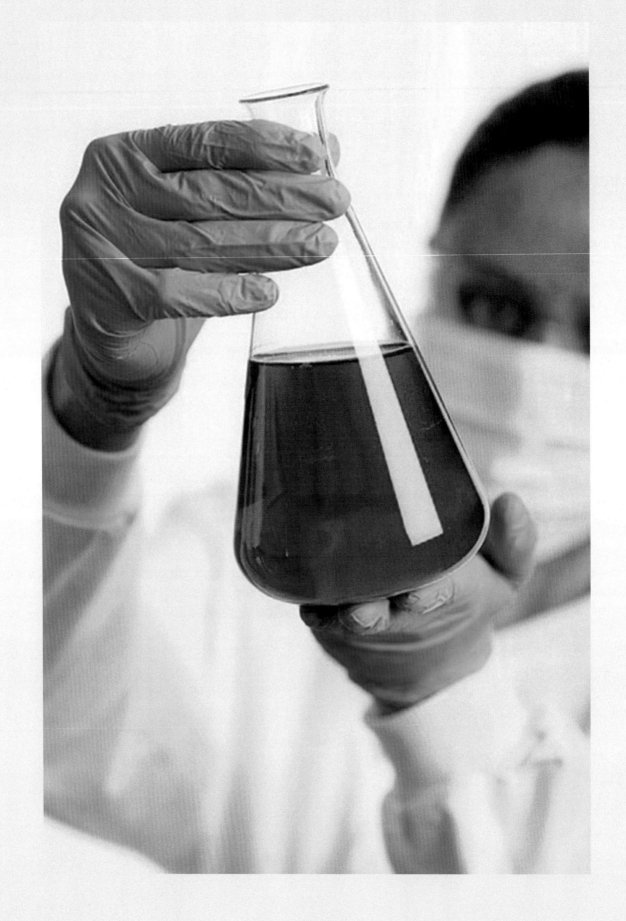

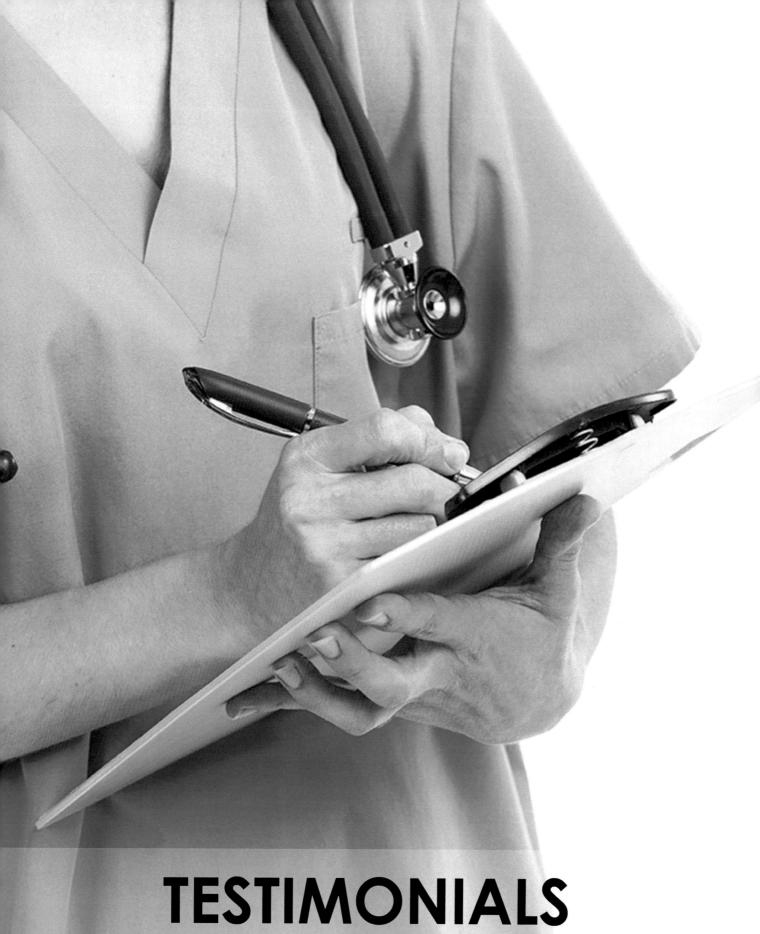

TESTIMONIALS

Dr Chris Strakosch
diabetic, cardiac, weight loss, cancer, improvement
Friday, 19 April 2013: Phone call 10:15 hours phone conversation

From: Kylie Harrison (registered nurse with registration number NMW000181573)

Witnessed by Mary Ann Meek
Confirmed Today 6 June 2013

On Monday, I called Greg, and he said, 'I think the cancer is gone'. He confirmed on Thursday's doctor's report.

White blood cell count from level 81 to level 55 (Greg's doctor wanted it at level 37). This count indicates a reduction in cancer cells.

Diabetes from 13 to 14.5 to 9, now 7 to 8. (Muscular spinal correction and cassia spice).

Pulse rate from 90, *now* 72–81; 71–82 (9 indicates cardiac improvement).

Stated blood pressure remains the same.

After Cranial Treatments and Stress Relief Initia
If this matter has not been dealt with in exercises, have 10 g of cassia per day.

Matter Private Dr Pia Lacovella (see Powerpoint end of book)

Phone call communication to Greg Farrell to assess his current physical condition after receiving treatment from Dr Gerhard Kempe, Thursday, 18 April 2013, for his heart condition/tachycardia and diabetes.

Baseline observation 15 March 2013 were as follows:

Height:	182cm
Weight:	196kg
Blood Pressure:	139/80
Pulse:	110bpm

Greg started the following changes (as of today):
- Nil dizziness (previously experienced constant dizziness)
- Nil chest pain (immediate after treatment aduring treatment)
- Chest pain prior was constant and described as uncomfortable
- Heart pulse rate decreased to 82 bpm
- Increased ability to sleep
- Increased mobility 100 per cent better
- Diabetes insulin reading has decreased from 13 to 9, now 7.2
- Weight loss (Greg is now 163 kg)
- Significant improvement in mental and physical capacities

Greg further stated he continues to lose weight (nutrition advice given by Dr Gerhard Kempe) and feels his diabetes is more manageable.

Greg has also received treatment from Dr Gerhard Kempe for a wound on his leg (impaired healing due to diabetes) with positive effect. In two days, swelling of leg has disappeared and the wound healed.

Lynn Noffke

Applied for a cleaning and work experience at the motel. She was in a bad health condition and limping, could not dance anymore. The stress in the eyes (pupil closed in, not surrounded by white of the eye), the limping—everything—pointed at a wreck, so I asked her whether she would welcome a health treatment prior to start. She laughed and said yes. The feet were 2 inches in height apart when lying on the front and knees bent. So after correction, the limping was gone. Sweat occurred on the forehead signs that there was a cardiac metre as well, and she fell asleep, losing time completely. A reaction often observed:

During intense corrections, the body just wants to repair and fall in alpha mode as the information newly provided including left-right condition requires to be in alpha mode.

Lynn Noffke (does not need a hip operation) works at Cleveland Visitor Villas Motel (phone 07 3286 5756) as assistant manager. Daughter, who also used the flu remedy, has no more migraine problems.

Alex (cardiac, kidney, blood pressure conditions) and Nora (blood pressure) work at Jaccaranda Cafe, 1/136 Gallery Walk Eagle Heights. Business owners who also used the flu remedy—now at Gallery Walk, Lick It, ice cream gelato and coffee shop.

Greg Farrel (diabetes, weight loss, cancer, cardiac) also used the flu remedy, which had amazing results that were demonstrated at Greenslopes Hospital, Brisbane Queensland.

David Noa (cardiac) is back to his rugby team and hairdressing.

Father Marce Singsong (kidney), of St Edwards Catholic Church Daisy Hill. Now back to the Philippines

Mary Ann Meek, Garden City Shopping Centre.

Empire Trade Barter Card Queensland had sold the topical remedies invented by Gerhard Kempe many years.

Members of the Lutheran Church, Mt Cotton, Queensland, were assisted with pneumonia.

Members of the Lutheran Church Mt Cotton (DV 1 www.healthyairtoday.com) with pneumonia asked, 'Gerhard, do you know what to do, my mother has pneumonia?' I answered, 'Easy, just have the portable DV 1 close to you and connected to electricity'. The pneumonia was gone in three days.
Pneumonia was gone in three days.
Three cases of pneumonia three times the same result; within three days, the sickness disappeared .
D V 1 was invented to create micro-organisms, free room air structures which benefit humans and plants and animals and devastate micro-organisms . Per ccm, more than ten million extra electrons on molecules and O_2, but no O_3 (ozone) is produced!
Ideal for surgery areas, intensive care, public counters, hospitals, and camps where refugees and soldiers are treated for injuries or infections.
The device is also used in mining camps and mobile hospitals.
For babies who cannot take medications and who suffer from whooping cough, a solution is found in the DV 1 as well.

ALEX ESCOBAR

Treatment for Alex Escobar included kidney, blood pressure, cardiac, weight loss, vitamin B complex, water plenty treatment.
'Gerhard, Nora and I talk about you as my angel and Nora's too. Your health recognition of my conditions, when we first met—just at my door—and the advice which I followed strictly together with your treatments were pillars for my health.
'I was close to death, obese, with high blood pressure, overworked, and doctors told me that I would require an operation soon.
'Nora's blood pressure is normal now as well after following your advice and without pharmaceuticals.
"You assisted me as well. Once, I could not lift my arms and you treated for cardiac improvement. And within thirty minutes, I could lift my arms without pain'.

LYNN NOFFKE

'Gerhard, I could dance again, and my doctor told me I do not require a hip operation anymore, and your migraine special topical medicine helped my daughter not to suffer migraines. As soon as they start, she applies your product, and the migraine is gone!'

MARY ANN MEEK

You are my angel that has assisted me in my health many times.
After an accident, Mary Ann could not find improvement. But with kinesiology, we started to learn and study it together. What an adventure through the paths of Eastern and Western medicine and with my combined knowledge of all both east and west, an airplane to fly through health. However, wealth has not yet been achieved with it.

ALEX ESCOBAR AND NORA

2006 – 13 Taillaroon Alex in 15 Tallaroon
Mobile 0466 272 504

ALEX ESCOBAR – CARDIAC

Sweat on the forehead. 'Gerhard, I came here, but I do not feel well, I have pain in my chest up to the shoulder, and I have to go home again', Alex said.
Gerhard asked, 'Alex, do you feel pain when raising your arms?' Alex answered, 'Yes'.
'Come over. Hop on the special treatment bed, and I will help you', Gerhard said.

Left-right condition—correction—muscular vertebrae re-arrangement in memory, cardiac test, and improvement and in memory.
 Alex said, 'Thank you, I feel well again—no more pain when I raise the arms. I can work now!'

DAVID NOAH – CARDIAC IMPROVEMENT

'I could mow all four properties in one day whereas before, I was puffing behind the mower
after a few steps, not able to mow one property in one day. Hey, Doctor, how are you? Did you realize what you did to me? I puffed behind the lawnmower with every step.

'I can get my pacemaker removed soon, and it can be used for another patient'.

David was a rugby player, and the diagnosis was cardiac from the very start. Once treated, the matter was instantly improved, and there were no more obstacles with his condition. It was perfect again.

To Whom It May Concern:

I take pleasure in writing this letter in regards to treatment Doctor Gerhard Kempe performed for not just myself but for my child whom suffered from severe migraines.

I had a bad hip and Dr Kempe performed a treatment which only seemed liked a 10 minute procedure (it actually took an hour) but it was so relaxing. Once the treatment was performed, I got off the bed and could walk without a limp and dance again. The doctors actually thought I would have to have a hip replacement. But thankfully I didn't after Dr Kempe's foot length treatment I do not have to go through a hip replacement.

My daughter whom also suffered with a bad migraines from a young age, at the age of nine, Dr Kempe gave me a small bottle to apply dab on her finger to her forehead and at the back of her neck when she felt migraine coming on. To my amazement, this worked. We had tried so many things and the doctors put her on Peractin and strict diet, this did not help. Today, my daughter aged nearly 13, has not had as many migraines and if she feels one coming on she applies the remedy herself.

I take this opportunity to thank Dr Kempe for all of his natural assistance and it is a relief to be pain free for myself and my daughter.

If anyone would like to know more please feel free to call me on 0468 436 404 (Australia)

Melinda Noffke
31 October 2013

GREG FARELL

'You, Mr Kempe, have helped me through my hardest times. No cardiac splint operation required. No cancer operation, weight loss 44kg without any malfunction but with improved capabilities. My diabetes is from 14 back to 7'.

What really had happened why all these persons enjoy such an enormous improvement in their health, with no operation, no pharmaceuticals (just less pharmaceuticals as directed by their doctors watching the improvement) is the Kempe Therapies, which I invented as all-in-one treatment, proved its values—non surgical cardiac improvements, muscular spinal correction and atlas correction placed into memory - left right condition correction placed into memory – dietetic advice - Holistic approach and www.healthyairtoday.com

TALA TUIALLI

From: Tala Tuialii
To: Dr Gerhard Kempe
Sent: Mon, 4 November 2013 04:59:01 +0800 (WST)
Subject: Witness report

Hi! I had the privileged to witness the work that Dr Gerhard Kempe did to some of our church members. Kempe's Health Therapy helped some of our church members including our pastor's wife who was quite ill at the time. The treatment worked and the people treated are well.
Tala Tuilii

From: CLEVELAND VISITOR VILLAS
To: westnet.com.au
Sent: Tues, 26 Nov 2013 08:21:52 + 0800 (WST)
Subject: Re: Flu Remedy

To Whom It May Concern
I have been taking Doctor Kempe's Flu Remedy for three years now and since taking it on daily, I have never got and signs of getting cold or any illness.

Before taking this remedy, I always used to get so sick in the winter months and now I am healthy all year round.

I highly recommend this to everyone, it is a natural remedy, with no toxins for your body.
If you wish to verify this please feel free to contact me on 0468 436 404 (Australia).

Kind Regards,

Lynn
Cleveland visitor Villas Motel & Shailer Park Garden Villas
Phone: (07) 3286 5756
Fax: (07) 3821 4169
E-mail: welcome@cvvmotel.com.au
        cvvspgv@gmail.com
        reservations@cvvmotel.com.au
Website: www.cvvmotel.com.au
Host: Lynn

ROSITA WHITE

Before I met Dr Kempe, I was suffering from a disease: a white, flaky like a dandruff that covers my whole scalp. I don't know if it is a psoriasis or eczema. I had this since I was young. I tried every possible medicine including different kind of shampoos as advised by many. The condition was so bad, my head was so itchy, flaky and it is infectious. It falls on my shoulder when I scratch it and it is very obvious ugly sight when I was wearing black dress. This disease also affects around my face, inside, out and the back of my ears. I sought the medical treatment from the General Practitioner and the doctor prescribed a medicine called, "diprosone or novasone lotion." A 30ml bottle with 0.05% betamethasone that cost more than A$ 20 a bottle, that will last only for one month. This medication works but the usage has to be continuous. If I stop using it the problem comes back with the very itchy flaky, white dandruff-like scalp disease. In the past I nearly lost my hair because this disease stops my hair from growing.

When I met Dr Kempe, he saw the white, flaky-like dandruff around my forehead and inside my hair (scalp). He advised me to use a mixture of salt and bicarb soda and soak myself in a bath and brush for seven minutes. So when I got home, I had a shower and forgot about the mixture of salt and bicarb soda. So what I did, after the shower, I made a mixture of the salt and bicarb and washed my hair again with this mixture and left without rinsing it overnight. What a miracle! Amazing! The next day all white, flaky head is *gone*! And my head scalp and hair is healthy again!

I can recommend Dr Kempe to anyone who suffers from any kind of diseases and conditions as he already treated many.

If you wish to contact me for further information, you can ring me on my mobile: 0450 622 138 (Australia 61)

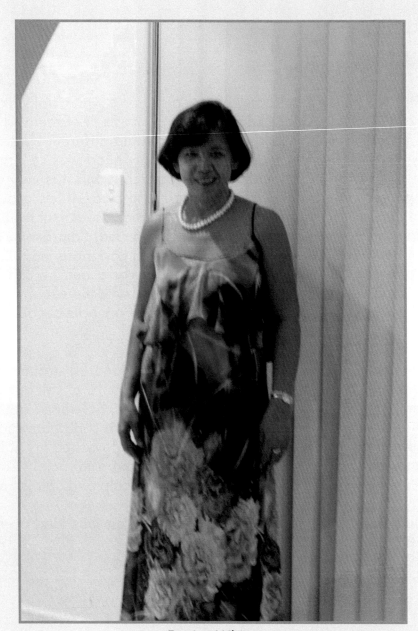

Rosita White

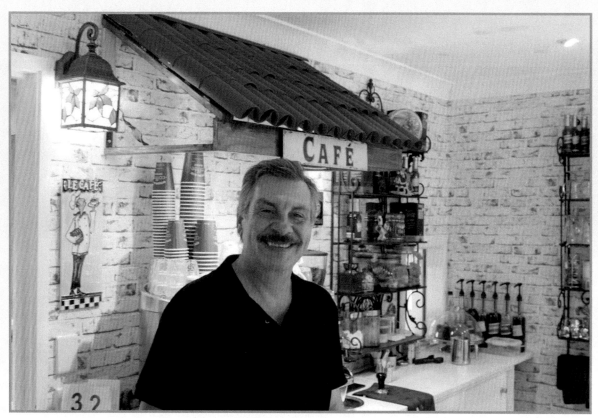

Alex Escobar

Lick it ice cream coffee and coffee shop Gallery Walk - Long Road Eagle Heights

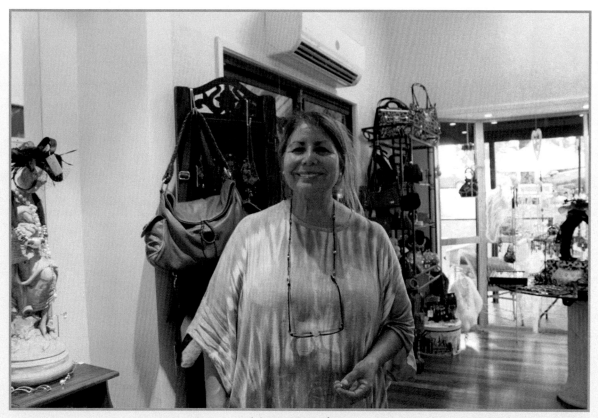

Nora Escobar

POWERPOINT PAGES

CARDIAC NON SURGICAL TREATMENT

VIRUS IN CARDIAC MUSCLE
TRY BISMUTH & SBC
IMPROVEMENT SUSTAINED

GF KEMPE(DR)
UNDISPUTED EVIDENCE
CLEAR MEASURABLE RESULTS

CORRECTION IN MEMORY

1 -1.5 HOURS INTENSE CORRECTION
25 MIN CHECK
30 MIN CORRECTION ON MPS

SAVE BILLIONS PHARMA& PACE MAKERS
&SURGICAL COSTS
IMMEDIATE CHANGE PULSE RATE
BLOOD PRESSURE ADAPTION
FULL POWER CARDIAC MUSCLE

D V 1

Susan.Rae@trade.qld.gov.au

EFECTIVE WIHOUT PHARMACEUTICALS AND WITH THEM www.healthyairtoday.com

ENVIRONMENT - ANSWERS FAST EFFICIENT SPEEDY

BEACH SOIL EROSION STOP

FIXED STRUCTURE PROVIDES
COUNTER WAVE

CLIENT PAY $ 1500 – 2500 PER QUARTER FOR 20 m Beach front property

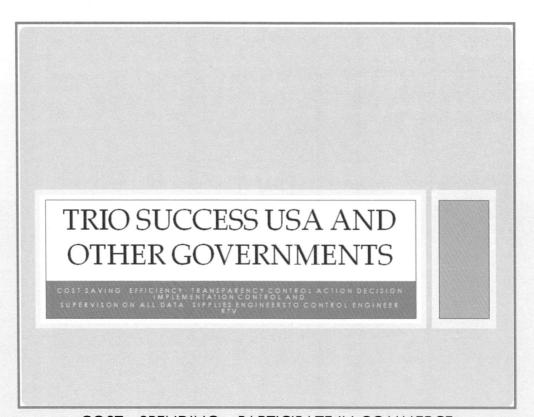

TRIO SUCCESS USA AND
OTHER GOVERNMENTS

COST SAVING EFFICIENCY TRANSPARENCY CONTROL ACTION DECISION
IMPLEMENTATION CONTROL AND
SUPERVISON ON ALL DATA SIPPLIES ENGINEERSTO CONTROL ENGINEER
RTV

COST - SPENDING – PARTICIPATE IN COMMERCE

GREENSLOPES HOSPITAL

PATIENT GREG FARRELL

KEMPE NON SURGICAL NON INVASIVE THERAPIES

DIABETES – WEIGHT LOSS – CARDIAC

IMPROVEMENT – DR STRAKOSCH

Psoriasis

Inside salt, zinc, Q 10, B complex, no wheat,
red beet root, greens, leaves, biofllavonoides,
pine -needles, selenium
Outside bath salt sodium bicarb; DV1;
+immune system-yoga-prayer; meditation

Inflamed ganglia connectivity or ganglia action with short-circuits

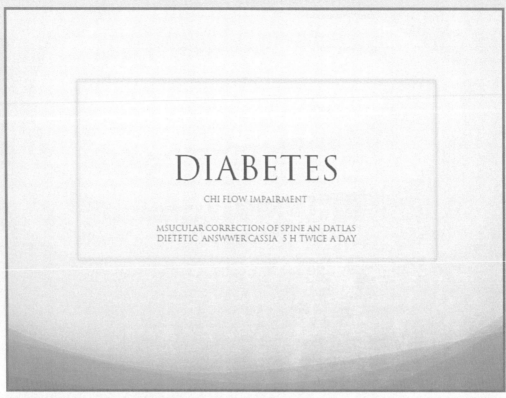

DIABETES

CHI FLOW IMPAIRMENT

MSUCULAR CORRECTION OF SPINE AN DATLAS
DIETETIC ANSWWER CASSIA 5 H TWICE A DAY

DIABETES - FARABLOC CAGE BUIDING SOLUTIONS – DIETETIC ANSWER – SPINAL CORRECTION AND OTHERS IN MEMORY

Skin Disorder

Zinc, Q 10,Calcium, B Complex, E
Cellery , apples, DV1, bath sodium bicarbonate water,
sinus relief, tintitus, virus, bacteria, salt, water
Mumps, Measeles, Rush, topical remedies, migraine,
headache, back pain, stress, addiction, athrithic, gout

Three layers of skin are subject to outside and inside attack, DV 1, pneumonia, whooping cough, stress, measles, rush, balance, fungus, fungi, bacteria, virus, viral attack

KINESIOLOGY COURSES VISITED 2005–2008

Touch for Health I, II, III, IV, and Synthesis

Cranial Kinesiolgy I, II, III

Brain Formatting

Chakra Metaphors

Neural Organisation Technique I and II

Neuro Spiritual Integration

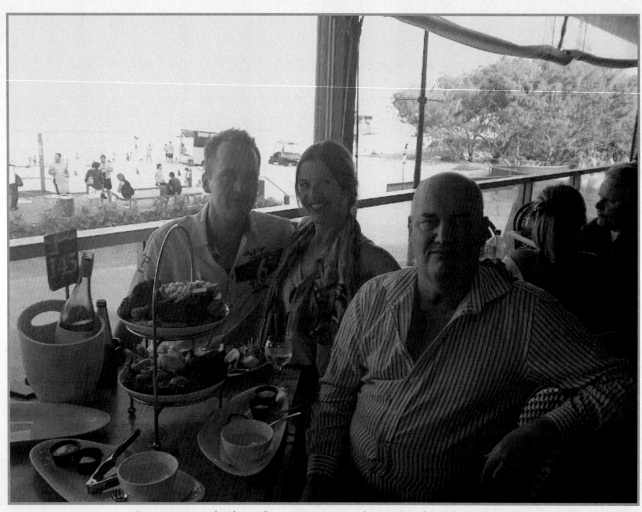

Son Konrad, daughter Katja and Dr Gerhard Kempe

Index

Printed in the United States
by Baker & Taylor Publisher Services